MW01231821

Diabetic Diet Crash Course

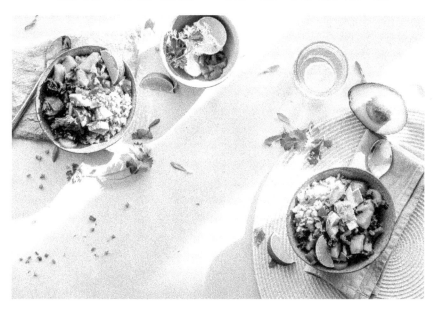

Definitive Guide To Delicious, Quick and Low-Budget Diabetic Diet Recipes To Eat Healthy, Weight Loss, And Change Lifestyle With Meal Plan For Beginners

Alice Louise Bayless

Table of Contents

5

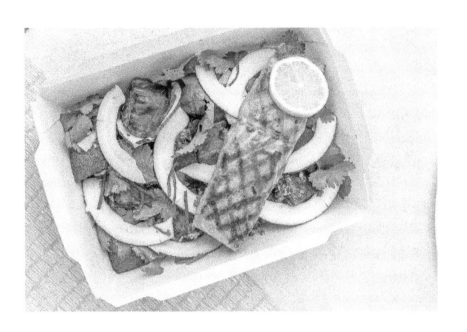

LET'S START!

Exercise For Diabetics

The most common types of diabetes are known as Type 1 and Type 2. The Type 1 diabetes, which is also known as adolescent diabetes, differs from Type 2 in the sense that the body will stop producing insulin altogether. Type 2 diabetes is normally diagnosed in older adults and occurs as the body stops producing enough insulin or the individual becomes resistant to their own body insulin.

No matter what form of diabetes it is, you'll lose your ability to adequately utilize sugar. The blood sugar levels will increase due to the body's difficulty in transporting sugar into the cells and out of the blood stream. There are several ways to lower your blood sugar levels, including diet, exercise, and medication.

As a whole, exercise is a very important part of diabetic management for both Type 1 and Type 2 diabetics. Those that have Type 1 will find regular exercise helps to maintain insulin sensitivity,
helps to prevent the accumulation of excess weight, and also increases the use of glucose by muscles. Although there is

really no way to prevent Type 1 diabetes, it is possible to prevent Type 2 diabetes.

The things to consider when you attempt to prevent the onset of Type 2 diabetes are regular exercise supplementation with vitamins and herbs that will help to prevent insulin resistance and proper control of weight.

Not only with exercise help directly with diabetic management by lowering blood sugar levels and maintaining insulin sensitivity, but it will also help minimize several of the complications that can occur in a diabetic individual. Research has shown that walking 30 minutes each day can diminish the possibility of developing Type 2 diabetes.

Almost all diabetics tend to develop circulatory problems and exercise can help lower blood pressure and improve circulation throughout the body. Seeing as how people with diabetes tend to have poor blood flow to their lower areas and feet, better circulation is a great benefit.

Even though there are risks associated with exercise, the potential benefits will outweigh the risks. Exercise does indeed lower blood sugar levels, so those with diabetes should measure their blood sugar both before and after they exercise. Since your body uses more sugar while you exercise and makes you more sensitive to insulin, there is a risk of blood sugar becoming too low and causing hypoglycemia as a result.

Whenever you exercise, it is important to let others know that you are diabetic. They should also be informed about what they should do in case of hypoglycemia. To be on the safe side, you should always carry candy or fruit juice with you to treat low blood sugar when it occurs.

During and after you have exercised, you should pay very close attention about how you feel, since rapid heart beat, increased sweating, feeling shaky, or hunger can signal that your blood sugar levels are getting too low.

With diabetic management and treatment, exercise is very important. Exercise will help with blood sugar control when the muscles use more glucose and the body becomes more sensitive to insulin.
Exercise will also help to prevent and minimize common diabetic complications which include heart problems, high blood pressure, and circulatory deficiencies.

If you are a diabetic, exercise should be part of your daily routine. You should always exercise at a slow pace and never overdo it. Also, you should be sure to exercise around people you know or at a gym, so there will always be people around you in case something goes wrong. Being a diabetic doesn't have to hinder your life or your performance, as exercise can help you get your life back on track and heading in the right direction - the healthy direction.

Tips for Revamping Favorite Recipes

Everyone has their favorite dishes, ones that mom or grandma used to make or new ones that you have discovered on your own. Once you have been diagnosed with diabetes, you may feel that you can never enjoy these dishes again (or not without harming your health).

But there are ways that you can change old family favorites keeping the flavor but reducing or eliminating the amount of sugar or carbohydrates they contain.

For most substitutions that you are going to make to your recipes, you are looking for ways to reduce the fat content. Here are some standards that you can use. When your recipe calls for:

- Whole milk try substituting with 2% or 1% instead
- Whole eggs try substituting with an egg substitute or use 2 egg whites for every whole egg called for in the recipe
- Sour cream use low fat sour cream or plan yogurt

- Baking chocolate try using cocoa powder mixed with vegetable oil (3 tablespoons with 1 tablespoon of oil will equal 1 ounce of chocolate)

In addition to the above suggestions, always use light or lower fat versions of ingredients.

Sometimes trial and error is necessary to get the recipe just right, but do keep trying the end result will be worth it when you create a cake or other dessert that you love and is diabetic friendly.

Alternately, you can purchase a diabetic cook book that is full of desserts to make that will work with your diet. This way you can create new favorites for you and your family to fall in love with. Don't feel that just because you are a diabetic you cannot enjoy variety in your foods.

Keep trying new things while keeping a close eye on your blood sugar levels to add new foods to your growing repertoire.

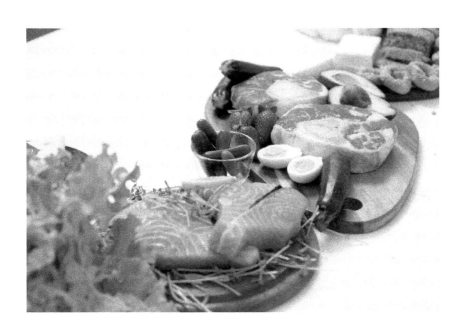

86 DELICIOUS
RECIPES

POLISH SAUSAGE STEW

Ingredients

- 1 can cream of celery soup

- 1/4 c. brown sugar

- 27 oz. can sauerkraut, drained

- 1/2 lb. polish sausage, cut in 2 inch pieces

- 4 med. potatoes, pared and cubed

- 1 c. chopped onion

- 4 oz. shredded Monterey Jack cheese

Direction

1. Cook sausage,potatoes, and onion until done.

2. Mix soup, sugar & sauerkraut, cook until blended.

3. Mix with other ingredients and top with cheese.

KRAUTRUNZA

Ingredients

- 1 link (approximately 1/4 lb.) German sausage

- 1 lb. ground beef

- 1 sm. head cabbage

- 1 med. onion

- Salt and pepper

- Yeast dough

Direction

1. Brown meats and add other ingredients, cook until tender. Serve

GERMAN SAUERKRAUT

Ingredients

- 1 can Bavarian sauerkraut, partially drained

- 1 apple, cored and sliced

- 1 onion, chopped

- or 3 slices bacon

Direction

1. Mix together and cook until all is tender.

POLISH BIGOS AND KLUSKI

Ingredients

- 2 lb. ground beef

- 3 tbsp. Crisco

- 2 c. diced green pepper

- 2 c. sliced onions

- 10 1/2 oz. can tomato soup

- #2 can tomatoes

- 3/4 c. water

- - 2 tbsp. salt

- 1/4 tsp. black pepper

- 1/8 tsp. red pepper (optional)

- 1/2 pkg. kluski noodles

Direction

1. Brown ground beef. Then add peppers, onions, cook until lightly sautéed. Cook noodles per package direction.

2. Add the rest of the ingredients and cook until well blended.

3. Mix sauce with noodles or let them put on their own sauce.

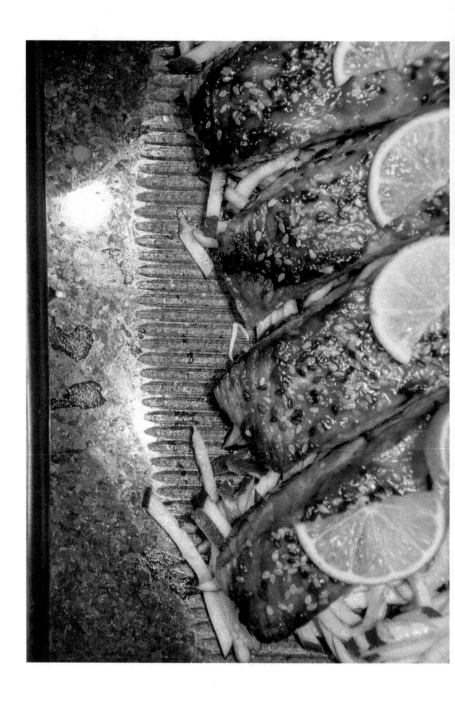

PATCHLINGS

- 5 c. flour

- 1 egg

- 1 tbsp. shortening

- 1 c. milk

Direction

1. Mix all ingredients together, drop on cookie sheet, and bake at 350 degrees for about 10 min.

WALNUT DREAMS

Ingredients

- ¼ lb margarine

- ½ c. + 1 tbsp brown sugar

- ½ c. chopped walnuts

- eggs (beaten)

- 1 ½ tsp baking powder

- 1 tsp vanilla

- ½ c. coconut

Direction

1. Mix all ingredients together and blend thoroughly.

2. Drop on cookie sheet , bake at 325 degrees until lightly brown.

SUGAR-FREE CHERRY OATS MUFFIN

Ingredients

- 1/4 cups unbleached flour

- 1/4 teaspoons baking powder

- 3/4 teaspoon baking soda

- 1/4 teaspoon lite (or regular) salt

- 2/3 cup all fruit black cherry jam

- 1/3 cup apple juice concentrate

- 1/2 cup cherry juice concentrate

- 1/2 to 3 Tablespoons canola or safflower oil

- 1/4 cup water

- egg whites or 1/3 cup egg white product

- 1 1/2 cups thin-rolled (quick) oats

Direction

1. Preheat your oven to 350 degrees.Sift dry ingredients together and set aside.

2. In a different bowl, lightly beat egg whites or eggbeaterss, and mix in all wet ingredients.

3. Mix liquid and dry ingredients,with a fork, just enough to moisten. Next, gently fold in oats and mix well.

4. Fill muffin tins 3/4 full, and bake at 350 degrees for 18 to 2⁵ minutes.

5. Check for doneness with a toothpick, if it comes out clean they're done. Cool about 10-15 minutes.

6. Serve warm or at room temperature. Makes 12 muffins

MOM'S WIENER SOUP

Ingredients

- 4 wieners

- 1 onion

- 1 qt. milk

- 1 1/2 tsp. salt

- 4 tbsp. butter

- tbsp. flour

- c. cooked, diced potatoes

- 1/4 tsp. pepper

Direction

1. Brown potatoes, wieners and onions in 2tbsp butter.

2. Mix milk, salt, pepper, flour and other 2 tbsp butter together, stir constantly until mixture boils and becomes smooth.

3. Then mix everything together in a soup pan or pot, cook until everything is hot, then serve.

GRANDMA LOE'S SKILLET CAKE

Ingredients
- 3/4 c. cake flour

- 1 tsp. baking powder

- 1/4 tsp. soda

- 1/4 tsp. salt

- 1 c. sugar

- 1/4 c. melted margarine

- 1 egg

- 1 tsp. vanilla

- Buttermilk

Direction

1. Put margarine in cup, add egg and fill cup with buttermilk (Blend with dry ingredients.) (beat) Before last line - sift flour baking powder, soda, salt and sugar into bowl.

2. Then beat with first mixture. Pour into skillet and top with topping.

--TUITTI-FRUITTI TOPPING--

- 1 c. drained fruit cocktail

- 1/2 c. brown sugar

- 1/4 c. chopped walnuts

- 1/4 c. margarine

1. Spoon fruit cocktail over top of batter, sprinkle brown sugar and walnuts on top of fruit cocktail, then drizzle with melted margarine

--ALMOND PRUNE TOPPING--

- 1 c. cooked prunes, halved

- 1/2 c. brown sugar

- 1/4 c. slivered almonds

- 1/4 c. margarine

MOM'S BEEF STEW

Ingredients

- 1/4 c. ginger ale

- 1 tbsp. red wine vinegar

- 1 can consomme soup

- Salt and pepper

- 1/4 c. flour

- 1 lb. lean stew meat

- 1/4 lb. mushrooms, sliced

- 1 med. potatoes, cut up

- 1 carrots, sliced

- 1 onion, sliced

Direction

1. Brown stew meat and sautee with onions and mushrooms.

2. Add all ingredients into pot and cook until meat is and vegetables are tender.

IOCOA EGG PANCAKES

Ingredients

- 8 eggs, whip hard

- 1 tsp. salt

- 1/2 c. milk or water

- 1 c. flour

Direction

1. Mix all ingredients and pour onto grill. Cook on each side until lightly brown.

DIABETIC BEEF PASTIES

Ingredients

--Crust—
- 3/4 tsp. Salt

- 1/4 c. plus

- 2 tsp. vegetable shortening

- 1 egg

- Water

Direction
1. Put flour and salt in mixing bowl. Cut in shortening.

2. Beat egg in a measuring cup.

3. Add water to make 1/2 cup, add to flour and mix until well moistened. Divide dough into 6 balls.

4. On lightly floured board, roll balls into circles between waxed paper. Then set aside.

--FILLING--
- 3/4 lb. coarsely ground beef (raw)

- 2 c. diced raw potato

- 3/4 c. diced raw carrot

- 3/4 c. diced celery

- 1 tsp. salt

- 1/4 tsp. black pepper

- 2 tbsp. water

Direction

1. Once all filling ingredients have been well mixed.

2. Spoon on to dough, and wrap around beef.

3. Bake at 350 degrees for about 10 – 15 min or until dough has become golden brown.

TUNA SUPREME

Ingredients

1   sm. can tuna, water-packed

- 3 hard boiled eggs, diced

- 1 c. American cheese, diced

- 1 tbsp. each chopped sweet pickles, mince onion, chopped celery and cut-up stuffed olives

- 1/2 c. mayonnaise or Miracle Whip

Direction

1. Mix all ingredients and serve on bread or lettuce leaf

DIABETIC SPICY MEATBALLS

Ingredients

- 1 lb. lean ground beef

- 1/2 c. chili sauce

- 2 tsp. prepared horseradish

- 1/2 c. minced onion

- 2 tsp. Worcestershire sauce

- 1/2 tsp. salt

- 2 tbsp. corn oil

Direction

1. Mix all ingredients well, roll into balls, and brown in corn oil. Drain on paper towels.

DIABETIC SPICY SAUSAGE

Ingredients

- 2 lb. extra lean ground pork

- 2 tsp. crushed dried sage

- tsp. freshly ground black pepper

- 1 tsp. fructose

- 1 tsp. garlic powder

- 1/2 tsp. onion powder

- 1/2 tsp. ground mace

- 1/4 tsp. ground allspice

- 1/4 tsp. salt

- 1/8 tsp. ground cloves

Direction

1. Mix all ingredients thourghly. Then make into patties and brown until done.

PORK CHOPS & STUFFING

Ingredients

- 5 pork chops

- box croutons, prepared to box directions, as stuffing

- 1/4 c. water

Direction

1. Brown pork chops, make sure cooked well. Serve with stuffing.

DIABETIC APPLESAUCE CAKE

Ingredients

- 2 c. raisins

- 2 c. water

- 3/4 c. oil

- 4 tbsp. Featherweight sweetener

- 2 eggs

- 2 c. flour

- 1 tsp. soda

- 1 1/2 tsp. cinnamon

- 1/2 tsp. nutmeg

- 1/2 tsp. salt

- 1/2 c. nuts (if desired)

- 1 c. unsweetened applesauce

Direction

1. Sift all dry ingredients together and set aside.

2. In a separate bowl mix all wet ingredients.

3. Mix wet and dry ingredients together and mix well, then fold in applesauce, nuts and raisins.

4. Pour in a greased and floured cake pan unless using a non-stick pan.

5. Bake at 350 degrees for 25 –30 minutes or until cake springs back when lightly touched in the middle.

BANANA BREAD

Ingredients

- 2 c. all purpose flour

- 1 tsp. baking soda

- 1 tsp. baking powder

- 1/2 tsp. pumpkin pie spice

- ripe bananas (mashed)

- 6 oz. can frozen orange juice

- eggs

- 1 c. raisins

- Nuts (optional)

Direction

1. Sift all dry ingredients together and set aside.

2. In a separate bowl mix all wet ingredients and mashed bananas.

3. Mix wet and dry ingredients together and mix well, then fold in nuts and raisins.

4. Pour in a greased and floured loaf pan unless using a non-stick pan.

5. Bake at 350 - 375 degrees for 30-45 minutes or when knife comes out clean

DIABETIC CHOCOLATE CHIP COOKIES

Ingredients
- 1/2 c. butter

- 1/3 c. brown Sugar Twin

- 1 egg

- 1 1/2 tsp. vanilla extract

- 1 1/3 c. all purpose flour

- 1 tsp. baking powder

- 1/2 tsp. baking soda

- 1/2 tsp. salt

- 3/4 c. skim milk

- 1/2 c. semi-sweet chocolate chips

Direction
1. Cream butter, brown sugar twin, vanilla and egg together. Sift all dry ingredients together in a separate bowl.

2. Add milk, dry ingredients and chocolate chips to creamed mixture.

3. Drop onto cookie sheet. Bake at 325-350 degrees for 7- 10 min. or until lightly brown.

WACHY CHOCOLATE CAKE

Ingredients

- 1/2 c. cake flour

- 1/4 c. cocoa

- 2 tbsp. granulated sugar replacement

- 1 tsp. baking soda

- 1/2 tsp. salt

- 1 c. water

- 1 tbsp. white vinegar

- 1/4 c. safflower or corn oil

- 1 tsp. vanilla extract

- 1 egg

Direction

1. Sift all dry ingredients together and set aside. In a separate bowl mix all wet ingredients.

2. Mix wet and dry ingredients together and mix well.

3. Pour in a greased and floured cake pan unless using a non-stick pan.

4. Bake at 350 degrees for 25 –30 minutes or until cake springs back when lightly touched in the middle.

APPLE PIE, SUGARLESS

Ingredients

- 12 oz. can concentrated apple juice

- 3 tbsp. cornstarch

- 1 tsp. ground cinnamon

- 1/8 tsp. salt

- 9 inch unbaked pie shell

- 5 sweet tasting apples, sliced

Direction

1. Mix all ingredients and bring to a boil.

2. When mixture starts to thicken remove from heat.

3. Pour into pie crust. Bake at 350-375 degrees or until golden brown.

APPLESAUCE COOKIES

Ingredients

- 1/2 c. all purpose flour

- 1 tsp. ground cinnamon

- 1/2 tsp. baking soda

- 1/4 tsp. allspice

- 1/2 c. quick rolled oats

- 1/2 c. raisins

- Nutmeats (Optional)

- 1/2 c. unsweetened applesauce

- 1 egg, beaten

- 1/4 c. shortening

- 1 tsp. vanilla extract

- 1/4 tsp. orange flavoring (optional)

Direction

1. Sift all dry ingredients (including oats) together in a separate bowl.

2. In a separate bowl mix applesauce, eggs, vanilla, orange flavoring (optional) dry ingredients and nuts.

3. Drop onto cookie sheet. Bake at 325-350 degrees for 7- 10 min. or until lightly brown.

DIABETIC OATMEAL COOKIES

Ingredients

- 3/4 c. vegetable shortening

- 1/2 c. Brown Sugar Twin

- 1/2 c. white Sugar Twin

- 1 egg

- 1/4 c. water

- 1 tsp. vanilla extract

- 1 c. all purpose flour

- 1 tsp. salt

- 1/2 tsp. baking soda

- 1 c. raisins

- 1 c. rolled oats, quick cooking or regular

Direction

1. Cream shortening, sugars, vanilla and egg together.

2. Sift all dry ingredients together in a separate bowl.

3. Add water, dry ingredients, raisins and oats to creamed mixture.

4. Drop onto cookie sheet. Bake at 325-350 degrees for 7- 10 min. or until lightly brown

HELEN'S LOW - CAL PECAN PIE

Ingredients

- 9 inch unbaked pie shell

- 3/4 c. egg substitute

- 3 tbsp. all purpose flour

- 1/3 c. plus 1 tbsp. plus 1 tsp. thawed frozen pineapple juice concentrate

- 1/4 c. sugar

- 1/4 c. dark corn syrup

- 2 tbsp. reduced calorie tub margarine, melted

- 1/2 tsp. vanilla extract

- 1/8 tsp. salt

- 1/2 oz. pecan halves

Direction

1. Mix all ingredients except flour and pecans and bring to a boil Now add flour and pecans.

2. When mixture starts to thicken remove from heat.

3. Pour into pie crust. Bake at 350-375 degrees or until golden brown on edges.

SUGAR - FREE SPICE COOKIES

Ingredients

- 2 c. water

- 1 c. raisins

- 1 sticks margarine

- 1 c. prunes, chopped

- 1 c. dates, chopped

- 1 egg whites

- 2 tsp. soda

- 1/2 tsp. salt

- 2 tsp. vanilla

- 1/2 tsp. cinnamon

- 1/2 tsp. nutmeg

- Dash cloves

- 2 1/3 c. flour, and maybe 1/4 more

- 1/2 - 1 c. nuts

Direction

1. Cream margarine, vanilla and egg whites together.

2. Sift all dry ingredients together in a separate bowl.

3. Add water, dry ingredients, raisins, dates, prunes and nuts to creamed mixture.

4. Drop onto cookie sheet. Bake at 325-350 degrees for 7- 10 min or until lightly brown.

DIABETIC BARS

Ingredients

- 1 c. dates
- 1/2 c. prunes
- 1 c. water
- 1 stick margarine
- 2 eggs
- 1 tsp. soda
- 1 tsp. vanilla
- 1/4 tsp. salt
- 1 c. flour
- 1/2 c. chopped nuts

Direction

1. Cream margarine, vanilla and egg together.

2. Sift all dry ingredients together in a separate bowl.

3. Add water, dry ingredients, dates, prunes and nuts to creamed mixture.

4. Spread in a cookie sheet pan. Bake at 325-350 degrees for 15-20 min. or until lightly brow

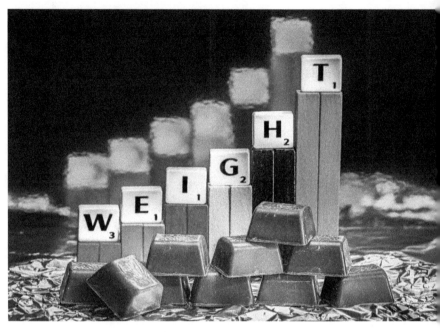

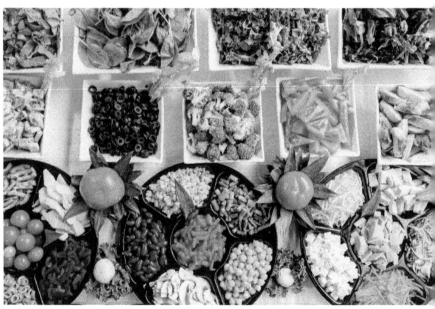

PICKLED FRENCH STYLE GREEN BEANS

Ingredients

- 1 can beans

- 1 tsp. pickling spice

- tsp. artificial sweetener

- 1/3 c. vinegar

Direction

1. Steam beans 5 minutes or less and strain.

2. Mix rest of ingredients and bring to a boil.

3. Strain to rid of spices.

4. If needed you can add vinegar or sweetener to taste. Pour over beans and let stand overnight.

ALOHA SEAFOOD DISH

Ingredients

- 2 lbs. fish fillets

- 1/2 c. pineapple juice

- 1/4 c. steak sauce

- 1 tsp. salt

- Dash of pepper

Direction

1. Place fish in single layer in shallow baking dish.

2. Combine remaining ingredients and pour over fish. Let stand 30 minutes, turn once. Remove fish, reserving sauce for basting. Place fish on Pam sprayed broiler pan.

3. Broil about 4 minutes, brushing with sauce.

4. Turn carefully and brush with sauce. Broil until fish flakes when tested with fork.

5. Garnish with lime wedges or pineapple if desired.

APPLE MAGIC

Ingredients

- 2 med. apples, pared, cored, coarsely chopped

- 1/2 tsp. cinnamon

- Artificial sweetener to equal 5 tsp. sugar

- 2 envelopes (2 T) unflavored gelatin

- 10 to 12 fluid ounces lemon-flavored dietetic soda

Direction

1. Preheat oven to 350 degrees.

2. In a deep, narrow, oblong pan arrange apples in layers. Combine 1 teaspoon cinnamon with sweetener to equal 1 teaspoon sugar.

3. Sprinkle some of this mixture over each layer of apples. Sprinkle gelatin over 10 fluid ounces soda to soften.

4. Add remaining sweetener and cinnamon; stir until dissolved. Pour mixture over apples; add remaining soda to cover apples. Bake at 350 degrees for 1 hour or until cooked throughout. While hot, refrigerate immediately, 4 to 6 hours or until set. Makes 2 servings.

APPLE TURNOVER

Ingredients

- 1 apple, peeled, cored and sliced

- 1 tsp. lemon juice

- 1 tbsp. water

- 1 slice white bread

- 1/4 tsp. cinnamon

- Artificial sweetener to equal 2 tsp. sugar

Direction

1. Cook sweetener, cinnamon, water, and lemon juice with apple Cook until tender.

2. Cool. Remove crust from bread.

3. Roll thin.

4. Place apple mixture on 1/2 bread.

5. Fold diagonally.

6. Moisten edges and press together with fork. Bake at 42! degrees slower until crisp.

APPLE/PEAR TUNA SALAD

Ingredients
- 1 med. apple or pear

- 1 (3 oz.) water packed tuna

- 1 tbsp. diced green pepper

- 1 tbsp. lo-cal French or Italian dressing

- 1 tsp. lemon juice

- Pinch of artificial sweetener

- Lettuce cup

Direction
1. Dice pear. Toss with tuna and green pepper.

2. Combine dressing, lemon juice, and sugar substitute.

3. Pour over salad and toss. Spoon into lettuce cup.

APRICOT UP-SIDE DOWN CAKE

Ingredients

- 12 frozen apricot halves, thawed

- 1/2 tsp. lemon juice

- 1/2 tsp. brown sugar replacement

- 1/4 tsp. cinnamon

- 2 slices white bread crumbs

- 1 tsp. baking powder

- Dash of salt

- 1 eggs, separated

- 1/3 c. granulated sugar replacement

- 1 tbsp. hot water

- 1/2 tsp. vanilla

Direction

1. Preheat oven to 350 degrees.

2. Combine apricots, lemon juice, brown sugar, and cinnamon. Spread on bottom of non-stick small baking dish.

3. Combine crumbs, baking powder, and salt. Beat egg yolks.

4. Gradually beat in sugar until yolks are thick and lemon colored.

5. Beat in water, bread crumb mixture and extract. Beat egg whites with a pinch of salt until stiff, not dry.

6. Fold into egg mixture. Spoon over apricots. Bake for 25 minutes or until cooked throughout. 2 servings.

BAKED APPLES

Ingredients
- Apples

- Cinnamon

- Artificial sweetener

- Non-sugar black cherry soda

Direction
1. Wash and core apples.

2. Slit and peel 1/3 of the way down.

3. Place apples in oven- proof dish and pour soda over them.

4. Sprinkle with cinnamon and sweetener.

5. Bake at 375 degrees until apples are tender.

BAKED BEANS

Ingredients

- 2 (16 oz.) cans French style beans

- 1 tbsp. dehydrated onion flakes

- 1 c. tomato juice

- 1 tsp. Worcestershire sauce

- 1 tsp. dry mustard

- Artificial sweetener to equal 12 tsp. sugar

Direction

1. Drain beans and empty into bowl.

2. Add remaining ingredients.

3. Mix lightly and turn into baking dish. Bake at 350 degrees for 45 minutes.

BAKED CHICKEN WITH APPLES

Ingredients

- 2 1/2 to 3 lb. chicken, cut up

- 1/2 tsp. salt

- 1/4 tsp. pepper

- 1 chicken bouillon cube

- 1/2 c. boiling water

- 1/2 c. apple juice

- 1 c. sliced fresh green beans, French style

- 1 c. diced peeled apples

- 1 tbsp. flour

- 1 tsp. ground cinnamon

- 1 oz. bread

Direction

1. Sprinkle both sides of chicken with salt and pepper.

2. Place chicken on a rack in a shallow open roasting pan.

3. Bake in hot oven (450 degrees) until browned, about 20 minutes.

4. Reduce oven temperature to 350 degrees.

5. Remove chicken and rack; pour off any fat from pan.

6. Return chicken to pan. Dissolve bouillon in boiling water.

7. Pour over chicken along with apple juice.

8. Stir in green beans.

9. Cover and bake 25 minutes. Stir in apple.

10. Cover and bake 10 minutes longer.

11. Meanwhile, in small saucepan mix flour with cinnamon.

12. Blend with 1 tablespoon of cold water.

13. Stir in hot pan liquid.

14. Cook and stir until mixture boils and thickens slightly.

15. Serve with chicken and vegetables.

BANANA CREAM PIE

Ingredients

- 2 c. skim milk

- 4 eggs, separated

- 4 packs artificial sweetener

- 1 tsp. banana extract

- 1 banana, sliced

- 1 packets unflavored gelatin

- 1 tsp. vanilla

Direction

1. Sprinkle gelatin in 3/4 cup cold milk. Heat remaining milk.

2. Add gelatin mixture and stir over low heat until dissolved.

3. Beat egg yolks, add to hot mixture stirring constantly.

4. When mixture thickens, add sweetener.

5. Remove from stove.

6. Add vanilla and banana flavoring.

7. Pour half of filling in 8 inch pie plate.

8. Place sliced bananas on top. Cover with rest of filling.

9. Meringue: Beat egg whites until frothy.

10. Add 1/2 teaspoon cream of tartar, 1 teaspoon vanilla.

11. Add 4 packs of artificial sweetener, 1/4 teaspoon nutmeg and beat.

12. Beat until stiff.

13. Pile on top of banana filling.

14. Put under broiler 1 to 2 minutes until golden brown.

15. Refrigerate 4 hours before serving.

BAR-B-Q MEATBALLS

Ingredients

- 1 lb. ground chuck

- 1/2 c. liquid skimmed milk

- 1 med. onion, chopped

- Salt & pepper to taste

- 1/2 c. diet catsup

- 1 tbsp. minced green peppers

- 1 tsp. prepared mustard

- 1 tbsp. vinegar

- 1 tbsp. minced onion

- 1 1/2 tbsp. Worcestershire sauce

- 2 packs Sweet & Low

Direction
1. Mix chuck, milk, onion, salt & pepper.

2. Make into balls.

3. Broil until brown (approximately 15 minutes).

4. Sauce: Mix catsup, green pepper, mustard, and vinegar.

5. Add minced onion, Worcestershire sauce, & Sweet'N Low.

6. Pour over meat balls. Cook covered for 15 minutes at 400 degrees.

BAR-B-Q SAUCE

Ingredients

- 1 can tomato juice

- 1 onion, chopped

- 1 tbsp. mustard

- 1 tsp. chili powder

- 1/4 c. vinegar

- Garlic powder to taste

- 1/2 tsp. paprika

- 1 tsp. Worcestershire sauce

- Sweetener, salt, & pepper to taste

Direction

1. Combine, bring to a boil then lower heat and simmer until thick as you desire.

BAR-B-QUE CHICKEN

Ingredients

- Chicken, boiled, skinned, boned, & chopped

- 1 can tomato juice

- 1 onion, chopped

- 1 tbsp. mustard

- 1 tsp. chili powder

- Sweetener to taste

- 1/4 c. vinegar

- Dash of garlic powder

- Pinch of oregano

Direction

1. Mix all ingredients, excluding chicken, to make the sauce.

2. Mix chicken and as much sauce as you like.

3. Simmer and eat on bread or without.

BROILED CHICKEN WITH GARLIC

Ingredients

- 2 1/2 lbs. chicken, quartered

- 6 cloves garlic

- 3/4 tsp. powdered rosemary

- Salt & pepper to taste

- Chicken bouillon

Direction

1. Rub chicken with 2 pressed garlic cloves, and rosemary.

2. Also rub with salt and pepper. Let stand 30 minutes.

3. Put chicken in broiler pan and coat top with bouillon.

4. Sprinkle with 2 slivered garlic cloves.

5. Add a little bouillon to pan. Broil turning when half done.

6. Coat top sides with bouillon and 2 more slivered garlics.

7. Baste with pan drippings.

BRUNSWICK STEW

Ingredients

- 3 oz. chicken breast

- 3 oz. ground chuck, cooked

- 12 oz. tomato juice

- 1/2 sm. onion or dehydrated

- 1 c. water

- 1 pkg. beef bouillon

- 1/2 tsp. red pepper

- 1/8 c. vinegar

Direction

1. Skin chicken and boil until tender.

2. Broil beef until brown.

3. Debone, chop, and blend chicken in blender.

4. Cook tomato juice, water, and onion slowly (30 minutes).

5. Add bouillon, pepper, meat, and vinegar.

6. Add salt and pepper to taste.

7. Cook very slow in a soup pot until thick or use a crockpot.

BUTTERMILK SHERBET

Ingredients

- 2 c. buttermilk

- Sugar substitute equal to 1/2 c. sugar

- 1 egg white

- 1 1/2 tsp. vanilla

- 1/2 to 1 cup crushed pineapple

Direction

1. Combine and blend well all ingredients except pineapple.

2. Pour into container.

3. Add pineapple. Freeze.

4. Stir occasionally until firm.

CABBAGE RELISH

Ingredients

- 5 lbs. cabbage

- 1 jar pimento

- 1/2 tsp. mustard seed

- 1 1/2 tsp. celery seed

- 4 tbsp. dehydrated onions

- 1 pt. white vinegar

- 1 tsp. salt

- Artificial sweetener to equal 2 1/2 cups sugar

- 1/2 tsp. turmeric

Direction

1. Grate or chop cabbage and pimento.

2. Mix remaining ingredients and heat mixture. When it comes to a rolling boil, cool. Pour over cabbage mixture.

3. Store in covered jars or container in refrigerator. Will keep several weeks. Taste better after it sets for a day.

CABBAGE ROLLS

Ingredients

- 6 lg. cabbage leaves

- 1/2 lb. ground chuck

- 1 tbsp. minced onion

- 1 egg

- 1 slices white bread

- Salt & pepper to taste

- Tomato sauce

Direction

1. Boil cabbage leaves in salt water for 5 minutes, set aside. Mix ground chuck, onion, salt, pepper, egg, and bread.

2. Carefully spread cabbage leaf. Roll up small roll of beef mixture. Secure with toothpick. Place rolls in boiler.

3. Pour tomato sauce plus a can of water over. Simmer about 45 minutes.

CABBAGE SALAD

Ingredients

- 3 c. shredded cabbage

- 1 tsp. salt

- 1 shredded turnip (2 oz.)

- 1 shredded carrot (2 oz.)

- 1 chopped green pepper

- 1/4 tsp. dill seed

Direction

1. Cover cabbage with salt.

2. Let stand for 45 minutes.

3. Wash and dry thoroughly.

4. Drain and squeeze all water out.

5. Toss with other ingredients.

6. Moisten with low-cal dressing.

CABBAGE SURPRISE

Ingredients

- 3 c. chopped cabbage

- 8 oz. ground chuck (raw)

- 1 tbsp. chopped onion

- 5 oz. tomato juice

- Salt & pepper to taste

Direction

1. Broil cabbage until tender, drain liquid and save.

2. Cook beef in Pam sprayed skillet, drain.

3. Drain meat on paper towels.

4. Combine ingredients and cook on low heat for 30 to 35 minutes.

5. If more soup is desired, add liquid from cabbage.

CABBAGE WITH TOMATOES

Ingredients

- 2 med. onions, sliced

- Artificial sweetener to equal 1 tbsp. sugar

- 1 med. cabbage, shredded

- 1 tsp. salt

- 1/2 tsp. caraway seeds

- 1 to 2 tbsp. vinegar

- 1/2 c. water

- 1 lg. tomatoes, peeled and chopped

- 1 tbsp. flour

- Bouillon

Direction

1. In deep saucepan, saute' onions in small amount of bouillon.

2. Saute' until soft and golden. Sprinkle with sugar. Add cabbage, salt, caraway, vinegar, and water.

3. Simmer, covered, over low heat for 30 minutes.

4. Add tomatoes and simmer, covered for 15 minutes more.

5. Mix flour with 2 to 3 tablespoons of pan liquid.

6. Make a smooth paste.

7. Stir into cabbage.

8. Cook, uncovered, stirring constantly until mixture thickens.

CARROT AND ORANGE SALAD

Ingredients

- 1/2 c. water

- 4 oz. grated raw carrots

- 4 oz. unsweetened orange juice

- tbsp. unflavored gelatin

- 1 tbsp. lemon juice

- Artificial sweetener equal to 2 tsp. sugar

- 1/4 tsp. salt

- Lettuce leaves

Direction

1. Soften gelatin in 1/4 cup cold water.

2. Add salt, sweetener, and 1 1/4 cups hot water.

3. Stir until dissolved. Add orange and lemon juice.

4. Set aside to stiffen slightly.

5. Add raw carrots to gelatin and pour into mold.

6. Make sure mold has been rinsed in cold water. Chill. Unmold on lettuce leaves

CELERY SALAD

Ingredients

- 4 c. slivered celery, sliced diagonally

- 2 heads Boston lettuce

- (12 oz.) yogurt

- 1 1/2 tbsp. lemon juice

- 1 1/2 tbsp. DiJon mustard

- 4 tbsp. finely chopped parsley

- Salt and pepper

Direction

Cover and cook celery in very small amount of boiling water. Cook for 3 minutes. Drain and cool. Arrange on lettuce cups. Mix yogurt, lemon juice, mustard, and parsley. Season to taste and pour dressing over celery.

CHEESE AND ONION CASSEROLE

Ingredients

- 8 oz. onions. sliced

- 4 oz. Swiss cheese, grated

- 4 eggs, slightly beaten

- 2 c. skim milk

- 2 tsp. salt

- 1 tsp. pepper

- 1 tsp. garlic powder

- 4 slices enriched white bread, crumbled, divided in half

Direction

1. Combine all ingredients except 1/2 of bread crumbs.

2. Combine in casserole dish; mix well. Top casserole with remaining bread crumbs.

3. Bake at 350 degrees for 25 minutes.

4. Bake longer if needed until cooked throughout. Makes 4 servings.

CHEESE CAKE

Ingredients

- 2 eggs

- 1 lb. Farmer's cheese

- 1/4 c. buttermilk

- 1 1/2 tbsp. liquid artificial sweetener

- 1 tbsp. lemon juice

- 1 tsp. vanilla

- 6 oz. cottage cheese

- 1/3 c. buttermilk

- 1/2 tsp. cinnamon

- 1 pkg. artificial sweetener

Direction

1. Blend eggs, Farmer's cheese, 1/4 cup buttermilk, then add liquid sweetener, lemon juice, and vanilla.

2. Pour into Pyrex dish and bake at 375 degrees for 15 minutes. Pour on cream topping and bake another 5 minutes.

TOPPING: Blend cottage cheese, buttermilk, cinnamon. Add sweetener and mix well

CHERRY BANANA DESSERT

Ingredients

- 2 c. cherry flavored sugar free beverage

- 1 envelope cherry flavored gelatin

- 1 sm. banana, peeled and sliced

Direction

1. Sprinkle gelatin over 1 cup of beverage.

2. Heat remaining beverage to a boil.

3. Combine with gelatin mixture.

4. Stir until gelatin is dissolved.

5. Refrigerate until thick. Add bananas and chill until firm.

BAKED CHICKEN DINNER

Ingredients

- 4 oz. chicken

- 1 egg

- 4 oz. cooked peas

- 1/3 c. dry milk

- 1 tbsp. dehydrated onion flakes

- 1 tbsp. green peppers, diced

- 2 tbsp. Worcestershire sauce

- 1/2 tsp. salt, seasoned

- 1/2 c. water

- 2 tbsp. pimento, chopped

Direction

1. Combine all ingredients. Bake at 350 degrees for 45 minutes.

CHICKEN LIVERS HAWAIIAN

Ingredients

- 1/4 c. liquid chicken bouillon

- 1/2 c. chopped celery

- 1/2 c. chopped onion

- 1/2 med. green pepper, sliced

- 12 oz. chicken livers

- 1 c. pineapple chunks

- 1 1/4 tsp. brown sugar substitute

- 1 tsp. salt

- 1 tbsp. cider vinegar

- Bean sprouts

Direction

1. Cook celery, onion, and green pepper in Pam sprayed skillet.

2. Cook over medium- high heat until crisp, about 5 minutes. Add chicken liver and cook 10 minutes.

3. Add chicken liver and cook 10 minutes.

4. Stir frequently. Add pineapple. Dissolve salt, sugar, and vinegar with 1/2 cup water. Add to skillet.

5. Serve on cooked hot bean sprouts.

CHICKEN LOAF

Ingredients

- 4 oz. chopped raw carrots

- 1 c. chopped raw celery

- 1 tbsp. dehydrated onions

- 1 sm. can pimento, chopped

- 4 tbsp. diet mayonnaise

- 1 1/2 c. water

- 1 pkg. or cubes chicken bouillon

- 1 envelopes unflavored gelatin

- 1 tsp. garlic salt

- 2 tbsp. mustard

- 1 tsp. lemon pepper

- 1 tsp. salt

- 1/2 tsp. pepper

- 16 oz. cooked, chopped chicken

Direction

1. Mix all ingredients except bouillon, water and gelatin.

2. Dissolve bouillon in 1 cup water. Dissolve gelatin in remaining 1/2 cup water. Add gelatin to boiling bouillon.

3. Add to mixture. Pour into loaf pan. Refrigerate. Unmold slice and serve.

CHICKEN SALAD

Ingredients
- 12 oz. sliced chicken

- 1/2 c. chopped celery

- 1/4 c. shredded carrots

- 1/4 c. lo-calorie salad dressing or mayonnaise

- 1/2 tsp. lime juice

- Salt & pepper to taste

Direction
1. Combine chicken celery, and carrots.

2. Stir dressing, juice, salt and pepper.

3. Pour over chicken mixture, tossing to coat well.

CHICKEN STEW

Ingredients

- 4 chicken breasts, stewed

- 1 (6 oz.) can mushrooms

- 1/2 med. head cabbage, chopped

- 1 med. onions, chopped

- Salt, pepper and garlic to taste

- 1 (12 oz.) tomato juice

Direction

1. To stew chicken, cover with water and pressure 15 minutes.

2. Remove chicken from water, add mushrooms, cabbage and onions.

3. Add salt, pepper, and garlic to taste. Add tomato juice and chopped chicken. Simmer for about 1 hour.

CHOCOLATE BAR

Ingredients
- 1/2 c. crushed pineapple, in own juice, drained envelope ALBA 77

Direction
1. Mix ingredients together. Make a tin foil pan the size of a large chocolate bar.

2. Pour ingredients into pan and freeze. When frozen, break into chunks.

CHOCOLATE CREAM ROLL

Ingredients
- 1 pkg. chocolate ALBA

- 2 eggs

- 1/2 tsp. cream of tartar

- 1/2 tsp. vanilla

- 1 pkg. Sweet'N Low

- 1/2 c. fruit juice

- 1 envelope unflavored gelatin

- 1/2 c. evaporated skim milk

- tbsp. lemon juice

- 1 tsp. vanilla

Direction

1. Blend ALBA, eggs, cream of tartar, and baking soda.

2. Add 1 1/2 teaspoon vanilla and Sweet'N Low. Blend in blender. Blend until smooth. Pour onto wax paper lined small cookie sheet. Bake at 350 degrees for 15 to 20 minutes.

3. Cool. Place on a slightly damp dish towel. Carefully peel away wax paper.

4. Cool. Spread with cream filling and roll up "Jelly-roll" style. Place the roll in freezer for storage.

5. Remove from freezer a few minutes before serving time. Slice.

CREAM FILLING: Mix fruit juice, gelatin, and milk. Add lemon juice, add 1 teaspoon vanilla.

CHOCOLATE PUDDING

Ingredients

- 1/3 c. chocolate Alba skimmed milk

- 1 egg

- 3/4 c. water

- Vanilla to taste

- Tart shells

Direction

1. Mix ingredients.

2. Cook until thick.

3. Serve in tart shells.

CHRISTMAS COLE SLAW

Ingredients

- 1/2 head green cabbage

- 1/4 head purpose cabbage

- 1/3 c. chopped onions

- 1/3 c. chopped green peppers

- 1/2 c. diet mayonnaise

- 1 tsp. salt

- 1 tsp. artificial sweetener

- 1/4 tsp. pepper

- 1 tsp. vinegar

- 1 tsp. lemon juice

Direction

1. Shred cabbage, chop onions and peppers.

2. Mix with other ingredients.

CRANBERRY GELATIN

Ingredients

- 4 c. fresh cranberries

- 1/4 c. cold water

- 20 packs Sweet'N Low

- 1 tsp. vanilla extract

- 1 1/2 c. water

- 1 envelope unflavored gelatin

Direction

1. Combine berries, 1 1/2 cups water, vanilla, and sweetener.

2. Combine in large saucepan. Bring to a boil. Simmer 1(minutes or until all berries pop.

3. Sprinkle gelatin on 1/4 cup water to soften.

4. Dissolve in hot cranberry mixture. Pour into mold and chil until set.

CREAMED SAUCE

Ingredients

- 1 box frozen cauliflower or fresh

- 1 (4 oz.) can stem and pieces of mushrooms

- 1/2 tsp. onion flakes

- 1/2 tsp. garlic powder

- Salt & pepper to taste

Direction

1. Cook cauliflower in water as directed.

2. Put in blender, using water it's cooked in.

3. Add mushrooms using water they are packed in.

4. Add onion flakes, garlic powder, salt and pepper. Blend until smooth.

CREAMY CHOCOLATE FUDGE

Ingredients

- 4 tbsp. diet butter

- 1/4 c. brown sugar replacement

- 1/4 tsp. instant coffee

- 1 envelope and 1/2 tsp. unflavored gelatin

- 1/4 c. cream flavored diet soda

- 2/3 c. nonfat dry milk

- 1 1/3 c. Ricotta cheese

- 1 tbsp. chocolate extract

- 1/2 tsp. vanilla

- 1 tsp. artificial sweetener (liquid)

- 1/2 tsp. brown food coloring

- 1 pkg. W.W. dried apples

Direction

1. Place margarine in a small pan over hot water to melt. Sif brown sugar and coffee very slowly into margarine.

2. Stir constantly. Soften gelatin in soda. Add nonfat dry milk Add a few drops more of soda if needed. The mixture needs to be paste like. Combine gelatin mixture with margarine mixture.

3. Stir constantly over hot water until thoroughly blended. Combine cheese, extracts, sweetener, and food coloring.

4. Mix well. Fold gelatin-margarine mixture into Ricotta mixture.

5. Pour into 8 x 8 x 2 inch pan. Refrigerate 2 hours. Freeze for firmer fudge. 20 squares.

CRUNCHY HAMBURGERS

Ingredients

- 1 lb. ground chuck

- 1 (16 oz.) can bean sprouts, drained

- 1 tbsp. Worcestershire sauce

- 1 tsp. salt

- 1 tsp. ginger

- 1/2 tsp. garlic

- 1/4 tsp. pepper

Direction

1. Combine all ingredients.

2. Divide mixture into 4 equal portions.

3. Broil on rack until cooled.

DELICIOUS SALMON

Ingredients

- 6 oz. salmon

- 1 tbsp. chopped green pepper

- 1/4 tsp. onion flakes

- 1/4 tsp. horseradish

- 1 to 2 tbsp. diet French dressing

- 1 oz. Swiss cheese

- 6 slices tomatoes

Direction

1. Mix first 5 ingredients well and divide into thirds.

2. Spread on 3 slices of toast. Add 1 ounce cheese and two slices of tomato.

3. Place under broiler until cheese bubbles.

DEVILED FISH BROIL

Ingredients

- 1 tsp. dehydrated onion flakes

- 1/4 tsp. Red Hot sauce

- 1/2 tsp. Worcestershire sauce

- 1/2 tsp. soy sauce

- 8 oz. uncooked fish fillet

- tbsp. prepared mustard

- 1/2 tsp. parsley, fresh, minced

Direction

1. Combine all ingredients except fish.

2. Mix well. Brush on both sides of fish.

3. Broil until fish flakes easily with fork.

DIET PIZZA

Ingredients

- 1 oz. bread

- 2 oz. cheese

- 1/4 c. mushrooms, sliced

- Pinch of garlic powder

- Pinch of oregano

- Tomato sauce or catsup (optional)

Direction

1. Put mushrooms on toast and cover with cheese.

2. Sprinkle with seasonings. Broil in oven until cheese is hot and bubbly.

DIETER'S DIP

Ingredients

- 1 (8 oz.) cottage cheese

- 1 (6 to 7 oz.) white tuna, packed in water

- 1 tbsp. chopped pimento

- 1 tsp. grated onion

- Salt & pepper to taste

Direction

1. Blend cottage cheese until smooth and soft.

2. Use blender or electric mixer. Drain and flake tuna.

3. Combine with cottage cheese and seasonings.

DIETER'S DRESSING

Ingredients

- 1 (10.5 oz.) can tomato soup, undiluted

- 1/2 c. tarragon vinegar

- 1 celery stalk, cut up

- 1 clove garlic

- 1 tsp. paprika

- 1 med. dill pickle

- 6 sprigs parsley

- 1 tbsp. Worcestershire sauce

- 1 tsp. prepared mustard

Direction

1. Place all ingredients in a blender in order listed.

2. Cover and run on high speed until vegetables are chopped.

DILLY TUNA SALAD

Ingredients

- 1 (20 oz.) can pineapple chunks

- 1 (6 oz.) can tuna, drained

- 1 c. cucumbers, sliced

- 1/3 c. imitation mayonnaise

- 1/2 tsp. seasoned salt

- 1/4 tsp. dill seed

Direction

1. Drain pineapple, reserving 2 tablespoons of juice.

2. Mix all ingredients except dill seed.

3. Line salad bowl with crisp salad greens.

4. Add above mixed ingredients. Sprinkle with dill seed.

DIPPIN PEAS SALAD

Ingredients

- 1 med. pear

- 1/2 c. cottage cheese

- 1 tsp. orange juice concentrate, thawed

- 1 to 2 tbsp. skim milk

Direction

1. Cut pear into wedges.

2. Place cottage cheese and orange juice in blender.

3. Blend until smooth, adding milk as needed.

4. Mixture should be very thick. Pour into small dish.

5. Use pear wedges to scoop up cottage cheese mixture. Makes 1 salad.

EGG SALAD

Ingredients

- 3 hard boiled eggs

- 3 oz. cottage cheese

- 1 tsp. mustard

- 1 tbsp. chopped onion

- 1 tbsp. dill cubes

- Crazy salt

- Pepper

- Finely chopped celery

Direction

1. Finely chop eggs. Mix all together.

2. Makes lunch for two. Good on sandwich with tomato.

3. Vary seasoning to suit your taste.

FRUIT 'N BREAD PUDDING

Ingredients

- 3 slices enriched white bread
- 1/2 med. bananas, peeled and sliced
- 1/2 c. sliced peaches with juice
- 1/2 c. cranberries
- 1/2 c. brown sugar replacement
- 1/2 tsp. ground cinnamon
- 1/3 c. water
- 1/2 tsp. banana extract
- 1/2 tsp. brandy extract
- Grated nutmeg (optional)

Direction

1. On baking sheet toast bread at 325 degrees until dry.
2. Cut toast into cubes. Combine toast cubes and fruits.
3. Dissolve brown sugar and cinnamon in water.
4. Add extracts.
5. Pour over fruit mixture, turn with spatula until well coated.
6. Let stand 5 minutes.

7. Turn again, scraping down sides of bowl. Place mixture in one quart size oven-proof casserole.

8. Bake uncovered for 30 minutes. Serve warm with dusting of grated nutmeg. Makes 3 servings.

FRUITED CHICKEN SALAD

Ingredients
- blended cottage cheese

- 2 tbsp. skim milk

- 1 tbsp. cider vinegar

- 1 tsp. grated onion

- 1 tsp. salt

- 1 med. green pear, cubed

- 1 med. apple, cubed

- 1 c. chopped celery

- Lettuce leaves

Direction
1. Mix celery, apple, pear, chicken, and salt until smooth.

2. Add onion, vinegar, milk, and cheese and toss.

3. Serve on lettuce leaves. Makes 3 sandwiches.

HERB SEASONED BROCCOLI

Ingredients

- 1/2 c. water

- 1 pkg. instant chicken broth and seasoning mix

- 1 c. broccoli spears

- 1/2 tsp. marjoram

- 1/2 tsp. basil

- 1/4 tsp. onion powder

- Dash of nutmeg

- 1 tbsp. margarine

- 1 tsp. lemon juice

Direction

1. Combine water and broth mixture.

2. Add broccoli, sprinkle with seasonings.

3. Cover, bring to boil, simmer 6 minutes until tender.

4. Drain. Divide on plates.

5. Top with margarine and lemon juice. 2 servings.

HERBED FISH FILLETS

Ingredients

- 1 lb. fillets

- 1/2 tsp. salt

- Dash of garlic powder

- 1/4 oz. drained chopped mushrooms

- 1/8 tsp. ground thyme

- 1/2 tsp. onion powder

- Dash of black pepper

- 1/2 tsp. dried parsley

- 1 tbsp. nonfat dry milk

- 1 tbsp. water

- 1/2 tsp. lemon juice

Direction

1. Sprinkle fish with salt and garlic powder.

2. Mix remaining ingredients and spread over fish.

3. Bake at 350 degrees for 20 minutes, until fish flakes with fork.

HOT OPEN FACED BEEF SANDWICH

Ingredients

- 1 tbsp. bouillon liquid

- 1 lb. lean ground beef

- 1 c. chopped green pepper

- 1 c. chopped onion

- 1 c. diet catsup

- tbsp. prepared mustard

- Artificial sweetener to equal 1 tsp. sugar

- 1 tbsp. vinegar

- Toasted bread

Direction

1. Brown beef in bouillon. Meanwhile, prepare the vegetable mixture. Combine remaining ingredients.

2. May prepare ahead to allow seasonings to blend. Add vegetable mixture to beef.

3. Turn heat on low and simmer covered for 30 minutes. Toast bread and spoon mixture over.

IMITATION BAKED POTATOES

Ingredients

- 1 (oz.) pkg. frozen cauliflower

- 1 packet instant chicken bouillon

- 1 tsp. fresh chopped parsley

- 1 tbsp. skim milk

- 1 c. water

Direction

1. Dissolve bouillon in water, add cauliflower, and cook.

2. Place in blender with other ingredients. Do not over blend.

LEMON-PINEAPPLE MOLD

Ingredients

- 1 envelope lemon gelatin

- 1 envelope lime gelatin

- 1 c. buttermilk

- 1 c. cottage cheese

- 1 1/2 c. boiling water

- 1 1/2 c. crushed pineapple

Direction

1. Dissolve gelatin in boiling water.

2. Mix cheese and buttermilk in blender until smooth. Pour into gelatin mixture. Add crushed pineapple.

3. Let set in refrigerator until firm.

MARY JO'S CONGEALED SALAD

Ingredients

- 2 envelopes unflavored gelatin

- 1 grapefruit, peeled and sectioned

- 1 c. boiling water

- 1 c. diet ginger ale

- 1/2 c. lemon juice

- 1 envelope Sweet'N Low

- 1 tsp. vinegar

- 1/2 tsp. salt

- 2 c. shredded cabbage

Direction

1. Soften gelatin in lemon juice.

2. Add boiling water stirring to dissolve gelatin. Add diet ginger ale, Sweet'N Low, vinegar and salt. Let chill.

3. When it begins to thicken, fold in grapefruit and cabbage.

MEAT LOAF

Ingredients

- 1 lb. ground chuck

- 1 c. evaporated skimmed milk

- 1 tbsp. dehydrated onion flakes

- 1/2 tsp. salt

- 1/4 tsp. pepper

- 1/4 tsp. dry mustard

- 1/4 tsp. sage

- 1/8 tsp. garlic salt

- 1/2 c. chopped celery

- 1 tbsp. Worcestershire sauce

Direction

1. Combine all ingredients and shape into a loaf.

2. Bake on rack at 350 degrees for 1 to 1 1/2 hours.

MEXICAN SUPPER

Ingredients

- 8 oz. ground hamburger (or veal)

- 1/3 c. chopped green pepper

- 1/4 head cabbage

- 1/2 c. onion

- 1 c. tomato juice

- Salt & pepper to taste

- 1 tsp. chili powder

Direction

1. Cook meat and green pepper in skillet.

2. In blender, blend cabbage and onion. Drain cabbage mixture. In saucepan, put tomato juice, cabbage and veal mixtures. Add salt and pepper to taste.

3. Add chili powder.

4. Cook until cabbage is done.

MOCK FRUIT CAKE

Ingredients

- 1/3 c. instant non-fat milk

- 1/4 c. chilled orange juice

- 1/2 apple, cored and chopped

- 3/4 c. red currants

- 2 tsp. lemon juice

- 1/4 tsp. cinnamon

- 1/8 tsp. maple extract

- 1/8 tsp. vanilla

- Artificial sweetener to equal 6 tsp. sugar

- 2 oz. bread, toasted and grated

Direction

1. Preheat oven to 350 degrees. Combine milk and orange juice in large bowl. Whip until stiff by hand or mixer.

2. Fold in remaining ingredients. Line loaf pan with wax paper. Pour ingredients into pan and bake 1 hour.

3. Remove and cool thoroughly. Divide in half.

NEXT--DAY TURKEY AND RICE

Ingredients

- 1 egg, slightly beaten

- 1/2 c. cooked, enriched rice

- 2 oz. cooked turkey

- 1/2 med. green pepper, chopped

- oz. onion, chopped

- 3/4 tsp. monosodium glutamate (optional)

- 1/4 tsp. soy sauce

- Pinch garlic salt

Direction

1. Cook egg in non-stick skillet over medium heat.

2. Cook until cooked throughout. Cut in bite-size pieces.

3. Add all remaining ingredients; mix well.

4. Cook until heated throughout. Makes 1 serving.

ONION DIP

Ingredients

- 6 oz. cottage cheese

- 2 1/2 tbsp. lemon juice

- 2 tbsp. buttermilk

- Dash of onion flakes

- 1/2 tsp. garlic salt

- Cake coloring for looks

Direction

1. Blend until creamy.

2. Serve with celery sticks or raw cauliflower.

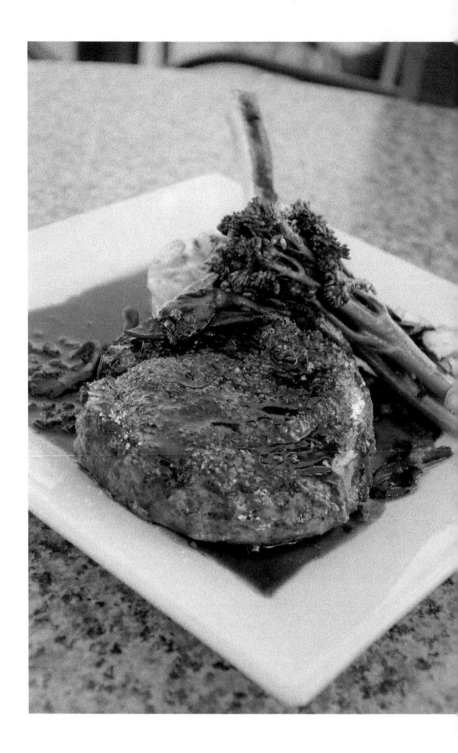

CPSIA information can be obtained
at www.ICGtesting.com
Printed in the USA
BVHW051602170821
614611BV00002B/200